ASTHMA IN CHILDHOOD

A.D. MILNER MD FRCP MRCS DCH
Professor of Paediatric Respiratory Medicine
Queens Medical Centre
Nottingham

Cartoons by *David Nathanson*

Churchill Livingstone ▦

EDINBURGH LONDON MELBOURNE AND NEW YORK 1984

CHURCHILL LIVINGSTONE
Medical Division of Longman Group Limited

Distributed in the United States of America by Churchill
Livingstone Inc., 1560 Broadway, New York, N.Y. 10036,
and by associated companies, branches and representatives
throughout the world.

© Longman Group Limited 1984

First published 1984

ISBN 0 443 02652 1

British Library Cataloguing in Publication Data

Milner, A.D.
  Asthma in Childhood.—(Patient handbooks)
  1. Asthma in children
  I. Title   II. Series
  618.92'238   RJ436.A8

Library of Congress Cataloguing in Publication Data

Milner, A.D.
  Asthma in childhood.

  (Churchill Livingstone patient handbook ; 16)
  1. Asthma in children—Handbooks, manuals, etc.
  I. Title.   II. Series
  RJ436.A8M54 1983   618.92'238   83-15238

Printed in Singapore by The Print House (Pte) Ltd

ASTHMA IN CHILD[...]

BRIDGEND GENERAL HOSPITAL

Nurse Training School and
Post Graduate Centre Library

This book can be borrowed for
14 days and may be renewed for
a further period, provided it
is not required by another
person.

WHEN BORROWING BOOKS, PLEASE
DATE AND SIGN ISSUE CARD AND
ENTER DATE ON THIS LABEL.

DATE	DATE	DATE
18 DEC 1990	. . . .	. . . .
03. AUG 1992	. . . .	. . . .
. . . .	. . . .	
. . . .	. . . .	
. . . .	. . . .	
	. . . .	

OTHER BOOKS IN THE SERIES

IN PREPARATION

PREFACE

This short book has been compiled in the hope that it will provide useful information for parents with asthmatic children. The questions used as a frame work have either been asked during consultation (often in my clinic) or were handed to me by the local Asthma Group. I am very grateful for their help. I also wish to extend my grateful thanks to Mrs Eileen Richardson for so patiently typing the drafts from my unintelligible hand writing.

Nottingham, 1983   A.D.M.

To *Jean Pierre*
the greatest of them all

CONTENTS

CONTENTS

1. WHAT IS ASTHMA?

A child is said to have asthma when he or she has recurrent attacks of coughing and wheezing which respond to asthma treatments. This rather bald statement does not take us very far, but in order to go further it is necessary to have a clear idea of the structure and function of the lungs.

The main role of the lungs is to provide a very large surface area (about that of a tennis court in an adult) so that the oxygen in the air can diffuse across into the blood, and then be transported to all parts of the body. At the same time, carbon dioxide, the waste or exhaust gas, is brought back to the lungs by the venous system so that this too can be diffused across the large surface membrane. The very large surface membrane is in the form of very small spheres, known as alveoli, each only 0.1 to 0.2 mm across, and too small to be seen without a microscope. At birth there are approximately 20 million alveoli. By the age of eight the adult number of three hundred million is reached and from then on the alveoli increase in size rather than in number.

If the alveoli are to be of any value it is obviously essential that the air within them is replaced continuously. This is achieved by drawing fresh air down a system of tubes. These tubes or 'airways' divide up to 26 times, becoming shorter and narrower on each division and eventually end in an alveolus. Much of the length of the airways is surrounded by a ring

1

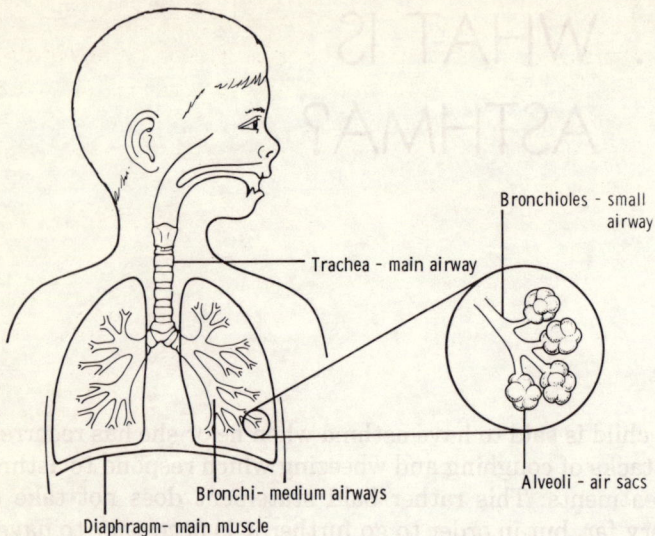

Bronchioles - small airway

Trachea - main airway

Alveoli - air sacs

Bronchi- medium airways

Diaphragm- main muscle

Fig. 1 The lungs and airways.

of smooth muscle which has a protective effect so that if an irritant and potentially dangerous gas is inhaled the smooth muscle will tighten, tending to close off the tubes and protect the delicate membranes beyond. All of us experience this to some extent on going out on cold, foggy nights, particularly in the industrial areas where the acid in the atmosphere converts a relatively benign fog into an unpleasant and potentially treacherous smog.

Children with asthma differ from their unaffected peers in that this tendency for the small muscles to tighten and constrict the airways, often referred to as bronchoconstriction, has been intensified so that conditions which rarely produce any symptoms in the healthy child then lead to difficulty in breathing, coughing and wheezing. The tightening of the muscles is accompanied by swelling of the inner lining of the tubes and by an out-pouring of secretions which make breathing that much more difficult. Breathing in is usually not too much of a problem as the airways are pulled open as the child sucks in air. Breathing out is a very different matter as the child tends to squeeze his airways closed as he tries to force the air out. This leads to wheezing on breathing out rather than on inspiration. It also produces a situation in which the lungs are pumped up and over-distended so that the child's chest, particularly the upper portion tends to be over expanded and the child sits with his shoulders held in an abnormally high position.

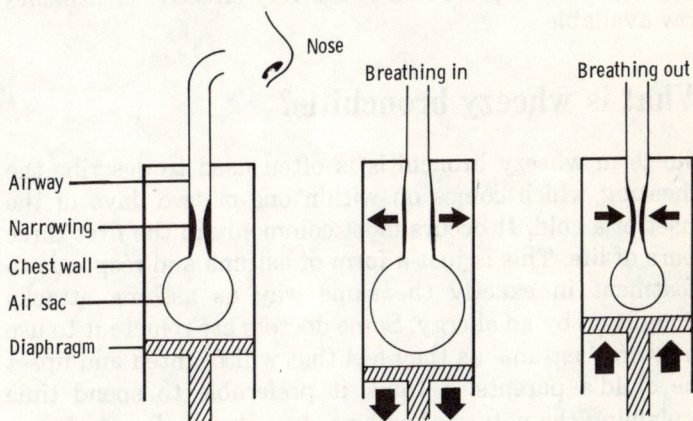

Fig. 2 Breathing in and breathing out in acute asthma attacks. The airways tend to be squashed on expiration.

There are many situations which can lead to bronchoconstriction and wheezing, indicating that asthma cannot be considered simply as an allergic problem. Rather, it is a condition in which the normal protective reflexes of the airway muscle and lining membranes are abnormally sensitive, leading to narrowing of the airways and producing attacks of coughing and wheezing. On this basis the incidence of asthma in childhood is approximately one in seven, or 15%. Most of these have only mild and very occasional attacks for which parents do not seek treatment.

Only about one in 30 or 3% are diagnosed as asthmatic and receive appropriate treatment. It is very important to stress that the large majority of those diagnosed as asthmatics have attacks which , although they are unpleasant, are not dangerous. The image that is often conjured up of a child who is effectively a respiratory cripple with greatly deformed chest, unable to join in games and almost totally isolated from his friends, is now extremely rare. We should never be frightened to accept that a child has asthma, as denying it will deprive him of the very effective treatments now available.

What is wheezy bronchitis?

The term wheezy bronchitis is often used to describe the wheezing which comes on within one or two days of the onset of a cold. It occurs most commonly in the first three years of life. This is just a form of asthma and responds to treatment in exactly the same way as asthma attacks brought on by an allergy. Some doctors are reluctant to use the word 'asthma' as they feel that will frighten and upset the child's parents. I think it preferable to spend time explaining the nature of asthma, how it will almost always respond to appropriate treatment and the excellent long-term outlook for many.

Why has our child asthma?

Even after lengthy discussions on asthma along the lines outlined above, most parents are understandably upset to hear that their child has asthma and want to know why their child should be affected. It is a question that doctors have considerable difficulty answering. There is no doubt that asthma occurs more commonly when parents or other close relatives either have asthma themselves or wheezed in childhood. This is largely due to genetic factors that the child has inherited. Having one asthmatic parent increases the likelihood of the child wheezing to about 20%. If both parents have asthma the risk approaches 30%. Conversely, the large majority of children born to asthmatic parents have no chest problems and over 65% of asthmatic children have a negative family history.

Acute bronchiolitis, a particularly unpleasant and severe viral lung infection which occurs in the first months of life, often renders the airways abnormally sensitive for some years. We have found that over 80% of children will wheeze in the months and years after the acute attack. This may in part explain why wheezing occurs so frequently in young children who have no apparent allergy problems.

There is no evidence that asthma is more likely to occur in 'sensitive or nervous children', nor that it is more common in bright children.

What makes our child wheeze?

Parents of asthmatic children frequently want to know what it is that brings on the wheezing attacks, hoping that there is a single trigger or allergy which, once identified, could be avoided and further attacks prevented. Unfortunately, asthma is rarely that simple.

By far the commonest cause of wheezing lasting for more than a few days is an infection of the nose and often the throat, in the form of a cold. This is particularly so in the first three years of life when wheezing and coughing are almost always brought on by viral infections. There is no practical means by which we can shield a child totally from these infections and, indeed to do so, might prove more dangerous in the long run as the child has to develop his own immunity. Antibiotics provide no protection and we have no effective vaccines against the many hundreds of viruses that the child is likely to meet. There is no evidence that the wheezing brought on by these viruses is in anyway representative of an allergic reaction. It is more likely that the inflammation accompanying the infection is itself sufficient to cause the airway muscles to contract and the lining to swell and weep.

Allergy undoubtedly plays an important part in wheezing attacks, particularly in the older child. A high degree of the population have an allergic tendency. Skin tests suggest that between 30 and 50% of all children have abnormal reaction to at least one substance. This is far in excess of the number who have wheezing attacks brought on by an allergy.

You could say that when a child has an allergy to something, his normal defence mechanisms have gone wrong. Our survival in our environment, containing as it does a wide range of viruses and bacteria, depends to a large extent on the presence of cells known as lymphocytes which

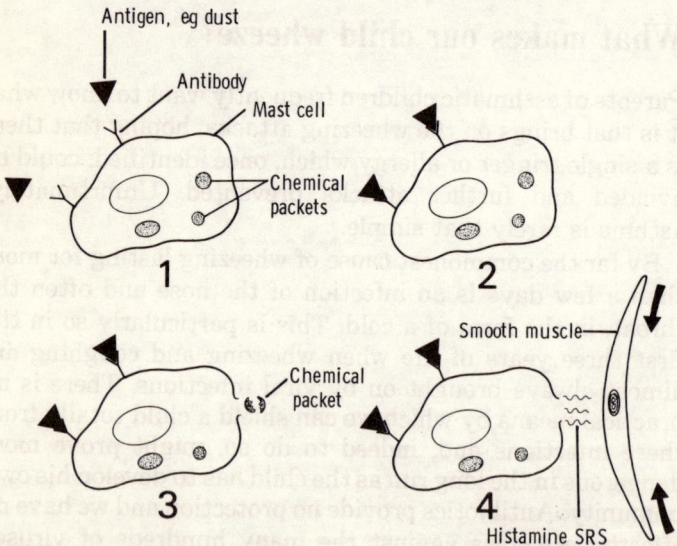

Fig. 3 The 'allergic' substances link in to antibody on the mast cell (1 and 2). This leads to the release of chemicals which cause the muscles to contract (3 and 4).

are scattered throughout the body. These cells identify viruses and bacteria as potentially dangerous invading organisms and produce proteins or antibodies which can destroy the invaders. There are several different forms of antibodies, each having a different role in the defence of the body. The exception to this is the IgE group which are not of known benefit but are produced in allergic people. They tend to form a coat on specialised cells lining the nose, airway passages and also the skin, known as mast cells. When the child comes into further contact with the proteins or chemicals which have stimulated the production of the IgE antibody, a reaction occurs between the two causing the mast cells to release a number of highly active compounds into the surrounding tissues. These include histamines and also slow-reacting substance (SRS). These chemical produce localised itching, swelling of the membranes and tightening of any smooth muscle in the proximity. If this occurs in the nose and eyes hay fever is produced, with nasal and eye itching, sneezing and running of both the eyes and the nose. In the skin eczema results. A smaller proportion of children will have asthma attacks. Why all the children who have an allergy with either hay fever or eczema do not get asthma is not entirely clear. It is possible that it is only those who have an abnormally sensitive airway as well who develop allergic asthma.

The range of substance or allergies which produce an asthma attack is very wide. Of particular importance are the scales and droppings of a microscopic creature, the house dust mite. This somewhat horrific creature lives on flakes of human skin which are most abundant in the bed. They thrive particularly well in damp conditions. It is likely that the house dust mite is a contributory factor in at least 50% of children with asthma. Many children also have a sensitivity to grass and tree pollen which are likely to make asthma worse during the late Spring and early Summer. A further exacerbation sometimes occur in the Autumn due to allergy to mould spores. Animal furs and feathers are the

D. House dust mite   Pollens   Animal fur

Moulds   Foods and drugs

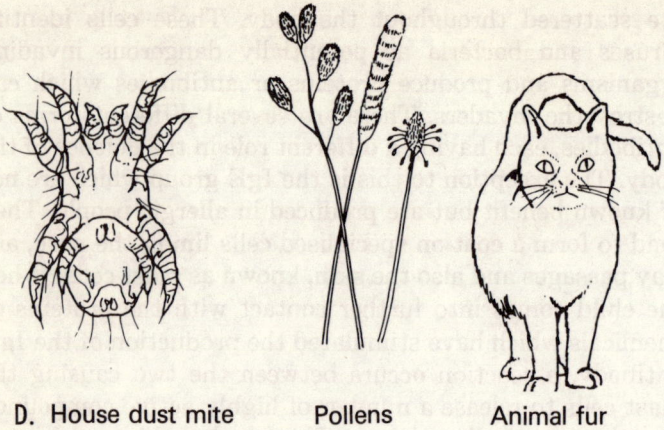

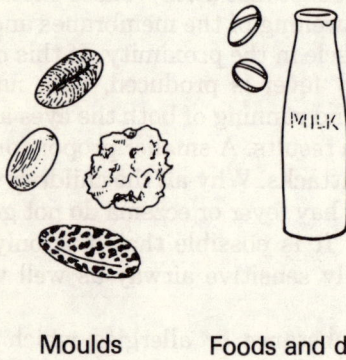

Fig. 4 Common causes of allergic reactions.

next most troublesome and it is not uncommon for parents to notice that the child wheezes and develops a hay fever like reaction and a skin rash on handling a friend's cat or dog. A variety of foods and drugs including cow's milk products, eggs and preservatives can also provoke attacks in a small number of children.

Wheezing and coughing after several minutes' strenuous exercise are almost universal in asthmatic children. These

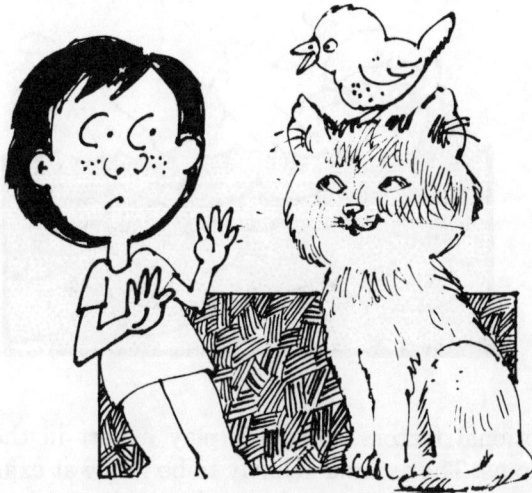

asthma attacks are fortunately short-lived, passing off within 15 to 20 minutes, even without any treatment but can be severe and distressing. Some children are so severely affected that they are unable to take part in even fairly gentle activities if they are not on appropriate treatment. We still do not fully understand the mechanism for this exercise induced bronchoconstriction but recent work has suggested that it depends on breathing dry cold air in to the airways rather than on the exercise itself. As one would expect it is more of a problem when the weather is cold and can be relieved by breathing through the nose, which is a very effective humidifier and heat exchanger. It also explains why asthmatic children have so little problem with swimming, a pursuit where the air immediately over the swimming pool is both warm and humid.

The asthmatic child is also likely to have wheezing attacks in any situation where the air is contaminated enough to cause coughing in even the healthy, unaffected person. These conditions include dust, smoke, fog, smog or other acid fumes. This probably just represents an increase in the normal protective mechanisms of the airways.

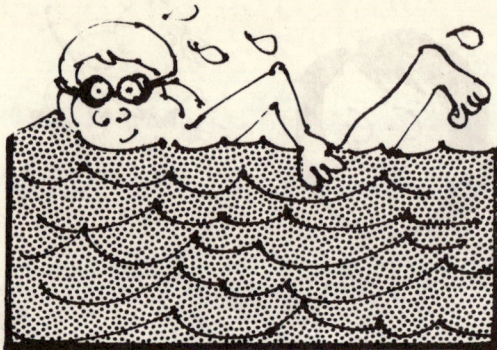

Emotional factors obviously play a part in the child's symptoms. The asthma is likely to be worse at exam times, when the child is excited or when there are emotional stresses and personality clashes at home or at school.

The list indicates the complexity of the disease; most factors, if not all, trigger wheezing attacks at some time or another. In the young child, i.e. under the age of three, viral infections are of an overriding importance, although some parents feel that weather conditions do have an effect. By the age of three to four years wheezing and coughing on exercise is present and often plays a major role in limiting the child's ability to join with his friends. Occasionally allergic factors bring on attacks in the first few years but for most this association does not emerge until the early school years, a time when emotional factors may also become important. Despite the emphasis given to allergic triggers, studies have shown that severe wheezing attacks lasting more than a few days are far more likely to be due to a viral infection than anything else throughout childhood. If the deterioration lasts for weeks or even months, stresses in the home or school should be considered.

In summary, it is well worth while trying to see whether there are one or two overriding problems which are largely responsible for the symptoms even though many parents are likely to find this a disappointing and rather fruitless exercise.

Does asthma damage the heart or the lungs?

Parents naturally become very concerned when their child has an asthma attack with coughing and wheezing lasting for hours. One particular worry is that the constant coughing may damage the child's lungs or even strain his heart. Fortunately this is not a problem. The child's heart escapes entirely unscathed and has little difficulty coping with even the most severe attack.

As already explained the lungs tend to increase in size during an attack as the air has greater difficulty escaping from rather than getting into the lungs. There have been worries that this would damage the lungs, leaving them perpetually over stretched like over-blown balloons. Even in the most severely affected this rarely ever occurs. Young children or those who have frequent and troublesome

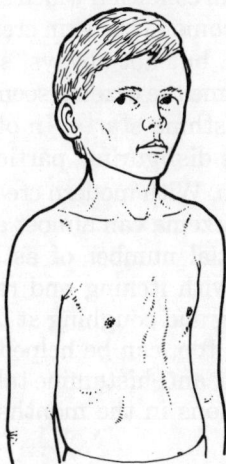

Fig. 5 Chest deformity in moderate to severe asthma.

11

attacks often have some chest deformity. This often takes the form of a prominence of the upper part of the chest and broad grooves over the sides of the chest with flaring of the ribs ends, which tend to stick out. These grooves which are several centimetres wide overly the attachment of the diaphragm, a large powerful sheet of muscle dividing the chest from the abdomen, and playing a large part in drawing air down into the lungs on inspiration. If the muscle has to work particularly hard it tends to pull the overlying bones in, particularly in the first years when the bones are relatively pliable. The chest deformity usually becomes less marked as the child gets older and the bones toughen. Even severe abnormalities will disappear eventually if the asthma subsides or becomes less severe.

Are there other diseases which are likely to occur with asthma?

Many children with asthma have previously had eczema. This is an itching skin condition which can affect all the body, but is most troublesome in the skin creases of the elbow and knee. Eczema often, but not always, starts in the first few months of life. In some the eczema seems to improve or even disappears as the asthma starts. In others it persists. The eczema can be quite disfiguring, particularly when scratching leads to infection. With modern creams, soap substitutes and medicines the eczema can almost always be kept under control. A substantial number of asthmatic children also develop hay fever with itching and red, discharging eyes, runny nose, sneezing and coughing at times when the pollen count is high. This, too, can be helped either by local anti-allergy preparations, anti-histamine tablets or by courses of desensitizing injections in the months before the pollen is released.

As already stated, asthma attacks rarely damage the lungs in childhood. Asthma persisting into middle age and later is more worrying and tends to merge with chronic bronchitis, responding less well to anti-asthma treatment. There are also a few children who have a gut sensitivity with vomiting, diarrhoea and abdominal pain in addition to wheezing. This pattern seems far less common in childhood than in adult life but it may be helped by omitting the item or items of foods which are responsible.

2. SHOULD OUR CHILD BE INVESTIGATED?

The majority of asthmatic children do not need any specific investigations, providing the asthma is relatively mild and responds well to standard treatment. Investigations are likely to be recommended if the child has to be referred to hospital or the asthma is causing worry and is proving difficult to treat.

What are blood tests for?

There are two blood tests that are likely to be arranged. For these, samples can be collected from a single finger prick or taken from a vein with a needle and syringe. The first is a routine test which few hospital patients escape, the full blood picture. The blood is examined to measure its red pigment content, the haemoglobin. In a child this will usually be 10–14 grams in every 100 ml of blood. A level below this indicated that the child is anaemic and may need medicine containing an iron salt or vitamins. Asthmatic children are, however, no more prone to anaemia than the rest of the population. A further part of the sample will be smeared onto a microscope slide and examined after appropriate staining so that the number of white blood cells can be assessed. Particular interest will be paid to white cells which contain granules which turn orange when stained, the eosinophis. The number of these cells increases in allergic conditions and in asthma it may exceed 1000 per cubic millimetre, over five times that found in non-allergic children. This then can be used as a marker for allergic problems. The second test involves measuring the level of the various groups of antibodies or immunoglobulins discussed earlier. Again the presence of high levels of the IgE group indicates that there is an allergic problem but will not differentiate between hay fever, eczema and asthma. It is also possible to carry out special tests to identify the nature of the IgE antibody and use the blood tests to characterise the substance to which the child is allergic. This is an expensive technique and usually provides little more information than can be provided by careful questioning possibly with skin tests.

What will a chest X-ray show?

A chest X-ray will be required if the child's symptoms are troublesome. Often the X-ray will be entirely normal. During an attack there will be further evidence that the lungs are over inflated and there may be some streaky shadows due to increased secretion in the airways. The main role of the chest X-ray is to confirm that there is no other problem present. Sometimes coughing and wheezing can arise because the child has inhaled a peanut or other object which is partially blocking off the bronchus. At other times part of the lung is found to be collapsed, possibly because of thick secretions. In these situations the sooner treatment is commenced with regular physiotherapy, if necessary proceeding to examination with a fibreoptic system under a light anaesthetic, the more likely the lung is to re-expand.

Should our child have skin tests?

Most children with troublesome asthma have skin tests at some time or another. These are often requested by parents

15

in the hope that they will reveal the allergy which is responsible for the child's wheezing. Unfortunately, this hope is rarely achieved. Skin testing is a safe and pain-free procedure. The aim is to introduce a very small amount of test substance into the child's skin. This is best achieved by

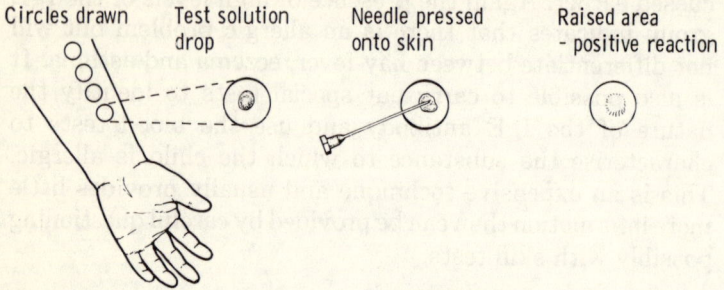

Circles drawn   Test solution   Needle pressed   Raised area
drop   onto skin   - positive reaction

Fig. 6 Skin tests.

placing a drop of the test substance onto the child's forearm and gently scratching the skin through the drop. It is usual to test the child's skin against at least six substances, including house dust mite, grass pollens and animal hair. A positive reaction is accompanied by a localised area of swelling which may range from only one millimetre in diameter, similar in size to nettle rash, to one to two centimetres not unlike a wasp sting. Although these have the appearance of stings, they only itch and are not painful and will subside within 30 to 60 minutes. The itching can usually be relieved quite rapidly by applying various creams. The relevance of the skin tests to the child's asthma is less easy to interpret. A positive test indicates that the mast cells within the skin are coated with antibodies against the test substance but as over 30% of non-asthmatic children have some positive skin test, correllation with asthma is not always good. If the child has a history of hay fever or wheezing when in contact with a particular animal or pollen that particular skin test is likely to be positive, but the reverse is far from always true.

However, the greater the skin reaction the greater the chance that there is an association. Thus, skin tests only give conclusive evidence on a sensitivity of the skin.

Some doctors use the nose as a test organ rather than the skin for investigating possible allergies. A positive test is indicated by sneezing and itching. Again there are many children who get hay fever and do not wheeze so that information is once more of limited value. The only way to be certain that a particular animal or plant is responsible for the wheezing is to measure the child's breathing before and after inhaling increasing concentrations of a solution of the suspected antigen and seeing whether an asthma attack is provoked. This is very time consuming as no more than one substance can be tested at each visit, and potentially a little dangerous as some children have a second and more severe asthma attack four to six hours after the first which does not respond easily to treatment.

How do lung function tests help?

Although we have a wide range of lung function tests available which give information on the state of the airways the two used most are the peak flow meter and the spirometer. The peak flow meter is a simple device which measures how fast the air can be forced out after a full inspiration and is measured in litres per minute. As the airways tighten the rate at which air can be driven out falls and so this provides a simple measure of airway constriction and can be used to assess the child's response to different treatments. The spirometer also comes in several forms but is essentially a device which measures how much air is forced out of the lungs, again after a full inspiration. This provides some information on the size of the lungs but in addition the spirometer can be used to measure how much air can be driven out after a certain time, usually three quarters or one second. As with the peak flow meter this volume, expressed in millilitres (ml) and litres and known as the forced expiratory

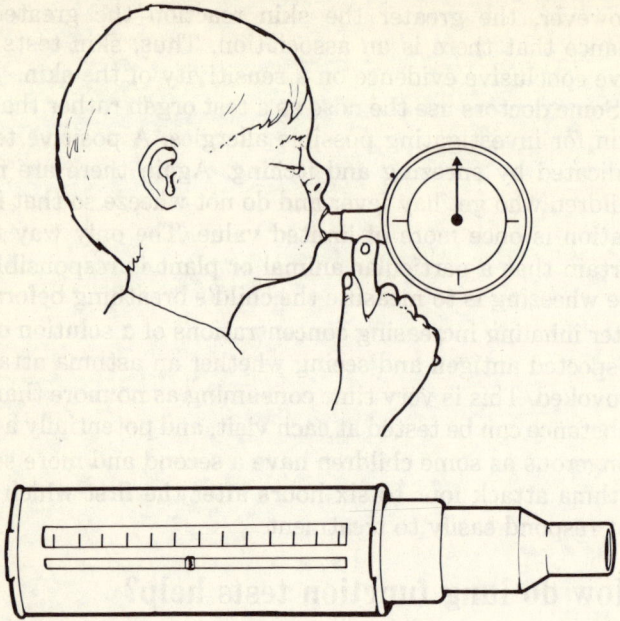

Fig. 7 The peak flow meter (top) and mini peak flow meter (bottom) for measuring lung function.

volume will be reduced when the airways are tight. Both these lung function tests are of very considerable value in the management of asthma. They can be helpful in diagnosis as a reduction in peak flow or forced expiratory volume which can be relieved by inhalation of an anti-asthma drug, such as Ventolin, confirms the presence of asthma. Subsequent tests give useful information on how the child is responding. If there is some doubt whether a particular form of therapy is helping, once or twice daily measurements of peak flow at home can build up a profile of the child's asthma. The peak measurements in the surgery or clinic also allow us to identify those children who have severe asthma and who need extra treatment.

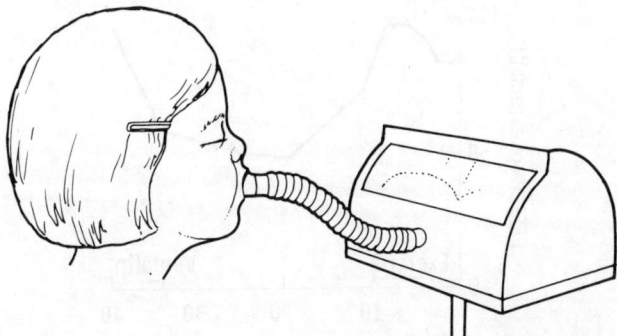

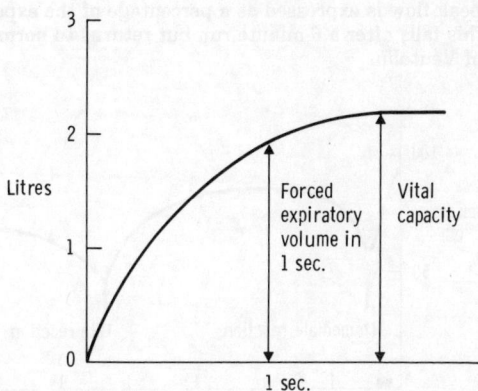

Fig. 8 The vitalograph. A spirometer for measuring the total volume of air the child can breathe out.

If the diagnosis of asthma is proving particularly difficult to clinch the child may be referred for more sophisticated tests. An example of this is the exercise liability test in which lung function is measured before and after 6 minutes of strenuous exercise. Children with asthma almost invariably show a fall in peak flow or forced expiratory volume of greater than 15%. Similar results can be achieved by giving the child inhalation of a naturally occurring substance, histamine, which itself plays a role in the onset of asthma at-

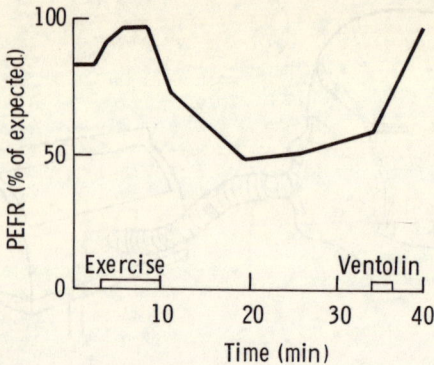

Fig. 9 The peak flow is expressed as a percentage of the expected for the child. This falls after a 6-minute run but returns to normal after an inhalation of Ventolin.

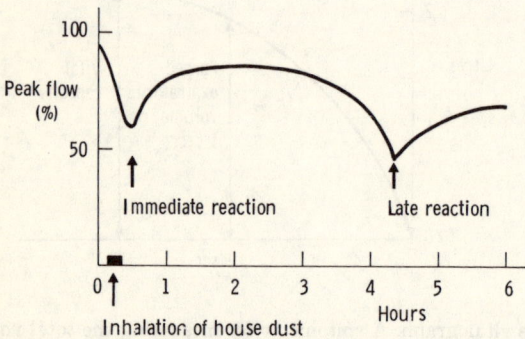

Fig. 10 The peak flow is expressed as a percentage of the expected for the child. The inhalation of house dust leads to a fall within a few minutes. A second fall may occur hours later.

tacks. The concentration at which bronchoconstriction first occurs provides information from the sensitivity of liability of the airway and again can be used to diagnose asthma. Finally, as already outlined, lung function can be measured after the inhalation of potential antigens, although this should only be carried out after taking special precautions.

3. WHAT TREATMENT ARE AVAILABLE? HOW DO THEY WORK?

There are now a bewildering number of drugs available for the treatment of asthma. These drugs can be divided into six separate groups, each acting by a different mechanism and having a different role to play. Many children with asthma will need only one form of therapy but sometimes drugs from two or even three groups can be used together with great benefit when symptoms are troublesome. These groups of drugs are the bronchodilator drugs (divided into Beta 2 stimulants and xanthene derivatives), the mast cell stabilisers, atropine derivatives, antihistamines and steroids.

What are bronchodilator drugs? How do they work?

The most common form of bronchodilator drugs are the so called Beta 2 stimulants. This group includes Ventolin (salbutamol) Brincanyl (terbutaline), Alupent (orciprenaline) and Pulmadil (rimiterol), Bronchodyl (reproterol) and Berotec (feneterol). Included in this group, although not strictly speaking Beta 2 stimulants as they have additional actions, are adrenaline and isoprenaline. These drugs all act directly on the smooth muscle of the bronchial tube, causing it to lengthen and relax. The mechanism of this is not fully

Table 1 Beta 2 stimulant drugs.

Trade Name	Proper Name	Preparation	Comments
Medihaler EP1	Adrenaline	Aerosol	Short acting. Stimulates the heart. Rarely used now
Medihaler 150	Isoprenaline		
Alendrin	Isoprenaline	Aerosol	
Ephedrine	Ephedrine	Tablets/syrup	Stimulates the heart. Becomes less effective with regular use
Alupent	Orciprenaline	Syrup, tablets Aerosol solution for nebuliser	Stimulates the heart slightly
Ventolin	Salbutamol	Syrup, tablets, slow release tablets, aerosol, rotacaps solution for nebuliser	Useful for night cough
Bricanyl	Terbutaline	Syrup, tablets, slow release tablets, aerosol solution for nebuliser	Useful for night cough
Bronchodil	Reproterol	Tablets/Aerosol	
Berotec	Fenoterol	Aerosol	
Pulmadil	Rimiterol	Aerosol	Very rapid onset but short acting. Has optional system activated by breath

understood but appears to be produced by stimulating the release of a chemical within the cell. This chemical is an enzyme known as cyclic AMP. Most of these drugs can be given by mouth as tablets or syrups but then take 20 to 30 minutes to reach their full effect. They act much more rapidly, within two to five minutes, if given by injection to a vein or if inhaled as a powder, a pressurised aerosol or a nebulised solution. As so often happens in asthma they are least effective when the asthma is at its most severe. They can be used to relieve most attacks and they are certainly very effective when given early. By and large they are remarkably safe. The oldest of the group, adrenaline and iso-prenaline, have now largely been discarded as these two drugs stimulate the heart and often produce headahces. They also have the disadvantage that they are broken down in the stomach and so cannot be swallowed. Even when taken by inhalation their effect only lasts for 30 minutes. The remainder of the group rarely have any significant effect on the heart, unless taken in very large doses when the heart rate may be increased. Their other side effect is a tendency to produce a tremor, a rapid almost imperceptable shaking of the hands which some find unpleasant. This is relatively rare in children and is of no significance. It passes off within 30 to 60 minutes.

The second bronchodilator drugs are the xanthene deriva-tives. These include various preparations of theophylline; Labophylline, Nuelin, Slo-phyllin, Theodrol, Aminophylline, Phyllocontin and other derivatives including Choledyl. These also cause relaxation of the smooth muscle but the mechanism is somewhat different. These all appear to pre-vent the normal reaction which breaks down the chemical cyclic AMP leading again to increased levels in the smooth muscle. These drugs can only be given by mouth or injec-tion. They are all too irritant to be inhaled. They are used in two different ways. First, by mouth as a regular therapy to control and prevent the onset of wheezing attacks. This has been made easier by the introduction of new slow release preparations in the form of special tablets and capsules containing mini-spheres which are slow to break down and release the active drug over 8 to 12 hours.

The second role for the xanthene derivatives, particularly aminophylline injections is to help relieve a severe attack which is proving to be particularly troublesome. Xanthene drugs unfortunately have rather striking side effects

Table 2 Xanthene (theophylline) derivitives.

Trade Name	Proper Name	Preparations	Comments
Choledyl	Choline Theophyllinate	Tablets	
Etophyllate	Acepifylline	Tablets, syrup, suppositories	
Cabophylline	Theophylline	Tablets	
Millophylline	Etamiphylline	Tablets, syrup	
Nuelin	Theophylline	Tablets, Syrup, slow release tablets	
*Phyllocontin Continuous	Aminophylline	Slow release tablets	
Phyllocontin Paediatric	Aminophylline	Tablets	
Silbephylline	Diprophylline	Tablets, syrup	
*Slophylline	Theophylline	Mini pellets in capsules	Contents of tablets can be emptied on jam etc
*Theodur	Theophylline	Slow release tablets	

* Only need taking twice a day. Can be taken in evening for night cough and wheeze.

tending to produce nausea and sometimes vomiting. They also increase the heart rate. The most worrying side effect only experienced if extreme over-dosing occurs is fits. Used properly these are very useful drugs which considerably help the young wheezy child.

There are other preparations, many of which have been on the market for decades, which contain several active ingre-

Table 3 Combination preparations (usually ephedrine and a xanthene drug).

Amesec	Cam	Expansil
Asmapax	Nethaprin Dospan	Taumasthman
Brontone	Franol	Tedral

dients, usually a Beta stimulent, particularly ephedrine, a xanthene drug such as theophylline and sometimes a sedative as well. Although used quite widely they are losing popularity to the newer and more effective drugs discussed above.

What are mast cell stabilisers? What is intal? What is zaditen? How do they work?

As already discussed there are mast cells present, particularly in the nose, lungs and skin which contain several asthma inducing substances, including histamine and slow releasing substance. There are now two drugs available which are claimed to stabilise the mast cells, that is render them less likely to release their contents on stimulation, whether this be by allergic factors, exercise and even emotion. These two drugs are Intal (sodium chromoglycate), and Zaditen (ketotifen). These two drugs differ strikingly. Intal is always inhaled in the treatment of asthma, either as a pressurised aerosol, powder or solution, while Zaditen is taken by mouth as a syrup or a tablet. The exact mechanism by which either of these drugs work is still in doubt. Intal is a very well established drug, is entirely safe, and appears to be totally without side effects, apart from a very occasional tendency to produce transient coughing, presumably due to the inhalation of the powder particles. Zaditen is still undergoing evaluation but may have a significant role, particularly in children with multiple allergies. This drug is related to the antihistamines which are so effective in hay fever and can produce drowsiness, although this has not proved to be a problem in children.

What is atrovent (ipratropium bromide)? What is atropine? How do these drugs work?

Although the main final pathway for inducing the smooth

25

muscle to contract is via the mast cell, there are also nerve fibres which can also cause bronchoconstriction. These are specialised nerves which form part of the automatic system and are not under our conscious control. They are particularly likely to induce tightness in the response to irritation in the airways and they may provide a route by which the emotions can influence the severity of asthma. It has been known for many years that atropine, a drug derived from Belladonna or Deadly Nightshade, can block these nerve fibres. Atropine, itself, has rarely been used for treatment of asthma in recent years as it has a number of side effects. These include an increase in the heart rate, and may dry up secretions making lung mucus difficult to cough up. In very large doses the child can become flushed and disorientated. For these reasons Atrovent (ipratropium bromide) has been developed which acts selectively on the smooth muscle nerves with little tendency towards other effects. This drug is usually given by inhalation. Its place in the treatment of childhood asthma has not yet been determined. It may well be found useful in the next few years.

What are antihistamines? What is phenergan, tavegil, piriton? How do they work?

As already stated histamine is one of the chemicals which are released from mast cells in response to allergies, exercise and possibly emotions and infections. We know that if an asthmatic child inhales even very small concentrations of histamine, he will inevitably wheeze for a few minutes. Antihistamines act by preventing histamine reacting with the smooth muscle. For this reason antihistamines have been given by mouth and occasionally by injection to children with asthma. Unfortunately, although antihistamines are very effective at controlling hay fever symptoms, they have so far been disappointing in childhood asthma.

One problem with all antihistamines, although to a varying degree, is their tendency to make the child or adult drowsy.

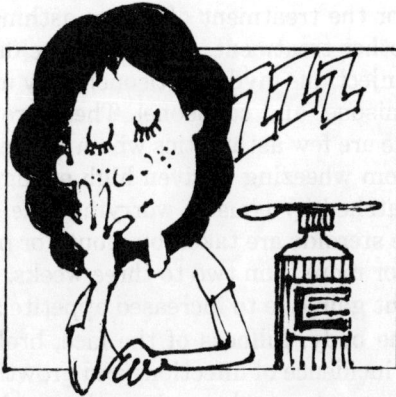

There is some evidence that antihistamines do have a useful effect on the lungs if high local concentrations are achieved. If given orally or by injection such large doses are required that the child will by then be soundly asleep! It is possible to get round this problem by inhaling the drug. Whether this form of treatment will be adopted in the future, again remains to be seen.

What are steroids? What is cortisone, hydrocortisone, prednisolone? What are becotide (bechamethasone), bextasol (betamethasone)? How do these drugs work?

All these are steroid drugs and are highly effective in asthma. How steroids work in asthma is not known. They do tend to relieve inflammation and are used in situations where the skin, gut, joints and even the arteries are affected in this way. They seemed to have a calming effect on the lungs, reducing the tendency for the smooth muscle to constrict, but do not themselves act as bronchodilator drugs. They take some hours to act and are used either as regular therapy or for the treatment of severe asthma attacks not relieved by other treatment. Some of these drugs can only be given by injections (hydrocortisone) or by mouth (prednisolone, prednisone, and cortisone). These are highly effective and there are few asthmatics who would not be entirely prevented from wheezing if given high enough doses. This benefit is matched by equally worrying side effects which emerge if the steroids are taken by mouth or by injection in large doses for more than two to three weeks. These effects include weight gain due to increased appetite and retention of fluid in the body, fullness of the face, broken veins, increase in the incidence of infections and growth retardation. Steroids in large doses also reduce the production of the body's own steroids which are essential in life. Sudden withdrawal of prolonged high doses of steroids can be dangerous and it is for this reason that children are usually issued with steroid cards to cover the unlikely event that they may be involved in an accident and taken to hospital unconscious. Side effects are very rarely seen if the drugs are taken over a period of a few days and so short courses given to cope with severe attacks of asthma should not cause any anxiety. Becotide and Bextasol, although steroids and presumably working by the same mechanism, are very different preparations and are a great deal safer. These drugs are inhaled into

Table 4 Inhaled steroid preparations.

Trade Name	Proper Name	Preparation	Comments
Becotide	Beclamethasone	Aerosol, Rotacaps Suspension for Nebuliser	Value not proven
Bextasol	Betamethasone	Aerosol	Stronger than Becotide

the lungs and as they do not dissolve in the body water remain there in close contact with the muscles and membranes. High local concentration can be produced even though the total dose is small and not taken into the body to any significant extent. For this reason a growth-suppressing effect and excessive weight gain rarely occurs unless very large doses are used. The only troublesome side effect has been for thrush to develop, identical to the yeast infection that is sometimes seen in the mouth of young babies. It is easy to treat and does not have any long term effects. Becotide and Bextasol have been very useful in the long term treatment but are not as powerful as the oral and injectible forms for acute severe asthma attacks.

4. HOW SHOULD WE USE THE VARIOUS TREATMENTS?

The easy answer to this question is to follow the advice of your doctor, but general guidelines can be given. As stressed in the previous section there are a large number of drugs available. Many of which can be taken in more than one form. My aim in this section is to provide information on situations in which these drugs can be used.

How should we use the ventolin, bricanyl, bronchodil, berotec and alupent? Should these drugs be taken by mouth as syrups or tablets or inhaled as pressurised aerosols, powders or nebulised solutions?

If the child has only occasional attacks of asthma which are not particularly severe it may be sufficient to give one of the above preparations in syrup or tablet form as soon as the coughing and wheezing starts. These will work within 10 to 15 minutes and reach the maximum effect by 30 to 60 minutes. The inhaled forms, however although rather more fiddly to take will act within one to two minutes and are generally a great deal more effective. There is no doubt that these drugs are more effective when given early before the tubes are blocked by secretions and are so safe that your child should not be denied the very considerable benefit that they produce. These medicines are also extremely useful for children who require other regular treatments and again should be given as soon as the asthma breaks through, producing coughing and wheezing. The inhaled preparations, aerosol or powder, provide excellent protection against asthma

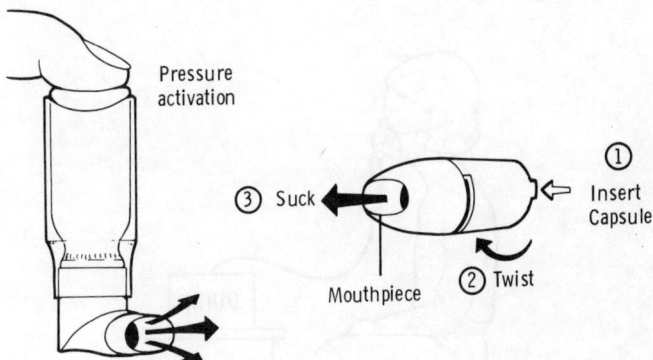

Fig. 11 The aerosol and rotahaler systems for inhaling drugs.

brought on by exercise and many children who would rarely by able to take part in games can join in with competitive sports if they have one or two puffs from the aerosol or inhale powder immediately before taking part. Your doctor may advise that you give your child this treatment regularly if the wheezing and attacks occur frequently. This is again entirely safe and the body does not 'get used to' the drug so that their effect is never reduced for future attacks.

One of the problems with all bronchodilator drugs is that their effect tends to wear off after four to six hours and so even if taken immediately before going to bed is likely to wear off in the middle of the night. This is a time when asthma symptoms are often at their worst, a fact which many parents with asthmatic children are only too aware. To get around this problem there are now a new generation of preparations appearing, for example, Ventolin spandets and Bricanyl slow release tablets which release the active ingredients slowly over 8 to 12 hours. Inevitably, however, these tablets are rather big and crunching or chewing the tablets eliminate their slow release characteristics.

The most effective method of administration is as a nebulised solution using an air compressor and nebuliser. This is now the first treatment all asthmatic children

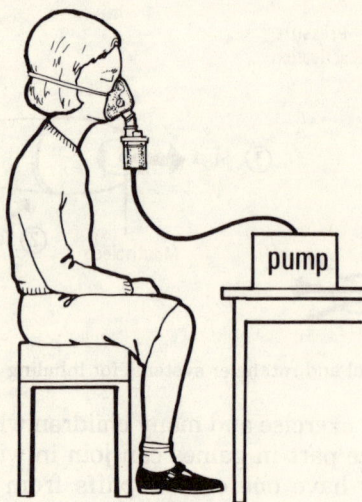

Fig. 12 The nebuliser and compressor in use.

receive when arriving at a hospital in a severe attack. Some general practitioners now have these systems and may bring them round to your home or make arrangements for inhalations at the surgery. If your child's asthma is severe or your child is under the age of four years the hospital may be able to provide a nebuliser for use at home, either as a regular or emergency treatment. The inhalation usually takes 5 to 10 minutes.

How should intal (sodium chromoglycate) be used?

Intal is usually prescribed when bronchodilator drugs are not controlling your child's asthma satisfactorily. As this is a preventive form of treatment it must be taken regularly, even when the child is apparently entirely well. Intal is now available in three forms. The commonest is as a powder which has to be inhaled from a device known as a spinhaler.

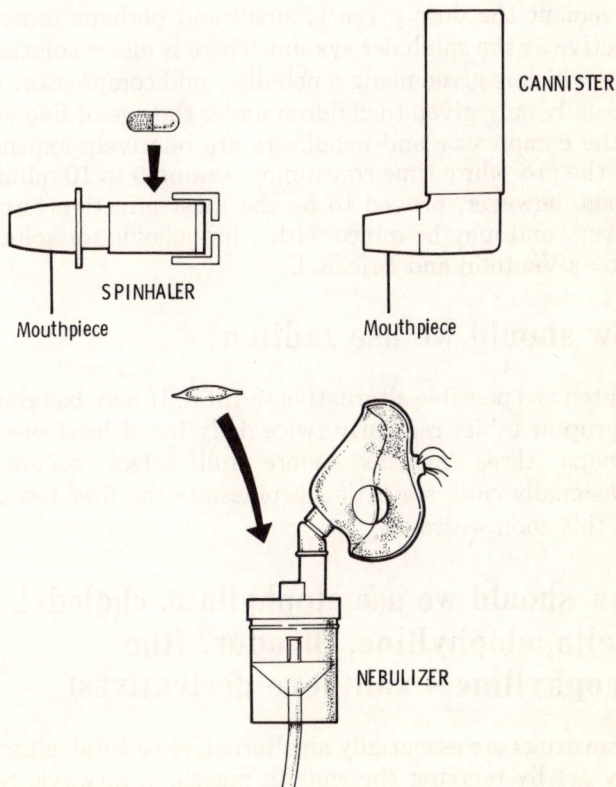

CANNISTER

SPINHALER

Mouthpiece

Mouthpiece

NEBULIZER

Fig. 13 The spinhaler, aerosol and nebuliser systems for inhaling Intal.

If your child is reluctant to use this device ask your doctor for a whistle 'attachment'. This whistle only sounds when the child sucks in. Very occasionally the powder produces some coughing. This can be prevented by inhaling a bronchodilator drug such as Ventolin immediately prior to the Intal.

The second and most recently introduced preparation is as a pressurised aerosol. Most children over the age of eight years can use these gadgets. What evidence is available suggests that although the delivery system is very convenient the dose given is small and perhaps is not as effective as the spinhaler system. There is also a solution of Intal which is given using a nebuliser and compressor. This is usually only given to children under the age of five years as the compressor and nebulisers are relatively expensive and the procedure time consuming, taking 5 to 10 minutes. It has, however, proved to be the most effective form of delivery and may be mixed with a bronchodilator solution, such as Ventolin and Bricanyl.

How should we use zaditen?

Zaditen is a possible alternative to Intal. It may be taken as a syrup or tablet regularly twice daily for at least one and perhaps three months before full effect occurs. It occasionally causes a little sleepiness in the first few days but this soon wears off.

How should we use etophyllate, choledyl, nuelin, slophylline, theodur? (the theophylline – xanthene derivatives)

These drugs are essentially an alternative to Intal, although they act by relaxing the smooth muscle of airways. Some doctors may decide to prescribe one of these drugs instead of, or even in addition, to Intal. This must again be taken by mouth on a regular basis. The newer preparations Nuelin, Slophylline, Phyllocontin and Theodur and continuous slow-release preparations and only need to be taken twice a day. They also provide an alternative to slow release Ventolin and Bricanyl for the control of coughing during the night. The dose required is fairly critical as high doses may cause some nausea and even vomiting. Many doctors start with a small dose and then increase this as necessary with the help of chemical analysis of blood samples. As before, the standard bronchodilator drugs such as Ventolin and Bricanyl can be taken in addition at times when break-through wheezing occurs.

Slophylline can be given to small children by emptying the contents of the capsule on to a suitable bribe. Those under the age of six years are unlikely to be able to take the other tablets.

How should we use atrovent?

Atrovent is currently only available in aerosols. Some doctors are now prescribing it to the older asthmatic child recommending that this is used at the same time as other bronchodilators drugs such as Ventolin and Bricanyl. This may be either regularly two to four times a day or just when your child has attacks of troublesome coughing and wheezing. There is some evidence that this form of combined treatment is better than either drugs alone.

How should we use the topical steroids, becotide and bextasol?

The topical steroids Becotide and Bextasol take some hours to reach their full effect and so must be taken on a regular basis, two to four times a day depending on response. These are more powerful drugs than either theophylline or Intal. Most of the younger children will have to use the rotahaler delivery system. Those over the age of eight may find the aerosol equally effective and less fiddly. Most doctors recommend that Intal is stopped if the child needs Becotide or Bextasol, but some seem to be helped by taking both preparations or a combination of Becotide and Theophylline When a child on a topical steroid has wheezing and coughing additional treatment with bronchodilator drugs such as Ventolin will often relieve the attack and, indeed, many doctors feel that any child who needs steroids should be on regular bronchodilator therapy. New topical steroids will be released on the market in the near future which will need only taking morning and evening. For younger children unable to use even the rotahaler there is a Becotide suspension which can be given by nebuliser. We are not sure how effective this is.

How should we use systemic steroids, prednisolone, prednisone, methyl-prednisolone and dexamethasone?

Systemic steroids are undoubtedly the most dangerous form of drug treatment we have and so it is essential that they are only taken exactly as your doctor advises. They are most often given in short sharp courses lasting three to seven days for attacks of asthma which are not controlled by the child's usual treatment, usually attacks brought on by colds, although other factors including allergy and emotional stress may be involved. The usual pattern is for the child to take one to two tablets three to four times a day up to 72 hours and then to reduce the dose day by day. A typical regime is shown in Table 5. Normally you will be advised to carry on with your child's standard treatment; otherwise there will be a tendency for the asthma attack to bounce back as the steroid dose is reduced. This type of course rarely has any side effects at all and can be considered quite safe. If an asthmatic child has several such attacks the child's parents

Table 5 Example of course of prednisolone for acute attacks of asthma not responding to normal treatment. The numbers indicate how many 5mg tablets have to be taken.

	Day 1	Day 2	Day 3	Day 4	Day 5
Morning	2	2	1	1	
Midday	2	2	1		
Evening	2	2	1	1	1

may be given one or more courses of tablets to start as soon as the asthma seems to be slipping out of control. This again is safe provided the attacks are relatively infrequent, for example, occurring less than once every three to four hours, If more frequent courses are required your doctor may decide to give the steroids as regular low-dose therapy, perhaps one to two tablets every other day. This is unlikely to stimulate your child's appetite and does not as a rule lead to any excessive weight gain or fluid retention. Any child on regular systemic steroid treatment will also need to take regular bronchodilator drugs and probably topical steroids as well. This will allow the dose of systemic steroids to kept to a minimum.

When should we use sedatives or antihistamines (piriton, phenergan, tavegil, anthisan)?

There is now a strong feeling that sedatives should never be given for acute attacks. Nevertheless, some children are given antihistamine preparations last thing at night. These help the child to sleep through and may reduce the coughing and wheezing early in the morning. The antihistamines, alas, have proved very disappointing in the treatment of asthma and are in general used less now than in previous decades.

5. WHAT OTHER TREATMENT IS AVAILABLE?

Although important, drugs are only part of the management of a child's asthma and many other aspects of treatment need to be considered.

Will a course of injections help our child's asthma? Can he be desensitised against his allergies?

Over the years, courses of desensitising injections have fluctuated in popularity and there are still quite a number of doctors who will be prepared to arrange a course of such treatment. The exact mechanism by which this therapy might work is not entirely clear, but the presumption is that injections of increasing strength will stimulate the body's own immune defence mechanism to produce antibodies in the blood stream. These new antibodies would then mop up the offending chemicals before they have a chance to combine with the IgE and set off the mast cell reaction. Evidence that this actually happens is slight. A further problem is that asthma is rarely due to a single allergy. There are few doctors who will now recommend the type of 'soup' injections which used to be prescribed based on the results of multiple skin tests.

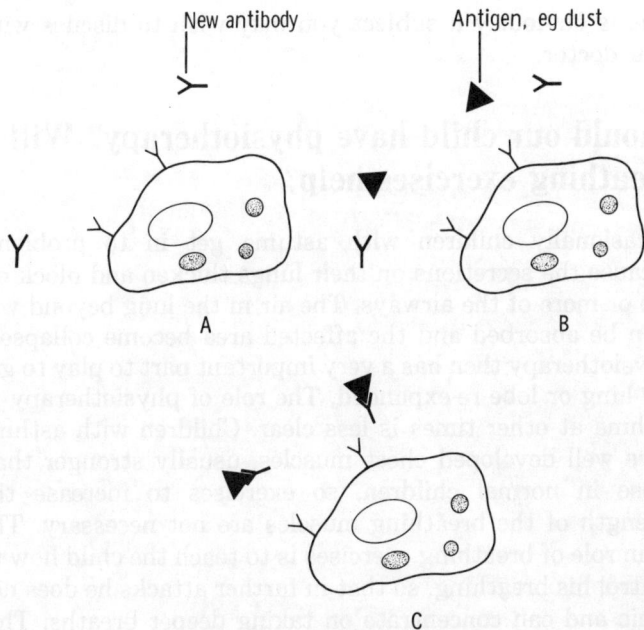

Fig. 14 'Blocking' antibodies. These new antibodies combine with the antigen before it can bind onto the IgE antibody on the mast cell wall.

There are undoubtedly some children who will seem a lot better for a period of months after a course of injections. Careful research has shown that children injected with water also often improve, although not quite as frequently, indicating the importance of the placebo reaction; the mind over the body influence, which is in us all and very potent in asthma. Desensitising injections are relatively painful and do sometimes cause local reactions not unlike large insect bites. Occasionally these produce a more extensive local reaction and on rare occasions can lead to a severe shock state which is potentially very dangerous. For this reason I feel that courses of injection are rarely indicated for asthma. They are much more helpful for hay fever and in that situation the benefit is considerable relative to the risk.

This is obviously a subject you may wish to discuss with your doctor.

Should our child have physiotherapy? Will breathing exercises help?

Occasionally children with asthma get in to problems because the secretions on their lungs thicken and block off one or more of the airways. The air in the lung beyond will then be absorbed and the affected area become collapsed. Physiotherapy then has a very important part to play to get the lung or lobe re-expanded. The role of physiotherapy in asthma at other times is less clear. Children with asthma have well developed chest muscles, usually stronger than those in normal children, so exercises to increase the strength of the breathing muscles are not necessary. The main role of breathing exercises is to teach the child how to control his breathing, so that in further attacks he does not panic and can concentrate on taking deeper breaths. This will limit the extent to which the tubes are narrowed by the child's own efforts and allow more air to pass in and out of the lungs.

Do ionizers help? How do ionizers work?

There are now a number of commercially available systems which generate minute particles of 'ions' which cause a negative electrical charge. It is claimed that when these installed in the child's bedroom the child will breath more easily. The theory behind these gadgets is that in animals, concentration of positively charged ions can cause airway smooth muscles to contract, reduce the production of mucus in the lungs and may even lead to pneumonia. It is assumed that negatively charged ions will have the opposite effect. Despite the fact that these devices have been around for a few years there is no good evidence that they do influence the severity of the child's asthma in any way. They are relatively expensive and cannot be purchased directly from the DHSS. If you do wish to use this technique it would perhaps be best to try and borrow one for a period of time to see whether your child does, indeed, improve.

Should we buy a humidifier for the bedroom?

Whether humidifiers are worth purchasing is rather more difficult. We know that breathing in dry air makes asthma worse and on these grounds it would seem sensible to install devices in houses with central heating systems where the relative humidity is low. Many children, particularly those with allergies, breath through their mouths rather than via their noses when asleep, bypassing the normal humidification process. It would not be unreasonable to feel that a humidifier might help in this situation. On the other hand the house dust mite, the microscopic animal which lives and breeds in the bed thrives best in moist conditions and so raising the humidity may increase the child's contact with this asthma-inducing foe. Although again there are no satisfactory studies on the subject it seems that some children benefit from increasing the humidity while others are made worse. If you are particularly anxious to try this form of treatment it would be worthwhile persuading the manufacturers to loan you a device over a two- to four-week period before committing yourself to perhaps unnecessary expense.

Is our child's asthma due to house dust mite? How dust-free should our house be?

Over 70% of children with asthma are allergic to house dust, particularly to the house dust mite. This rather horrific looking animal lives on shed human skin scales and so is found in most abundance in the bed and bedroom. You may

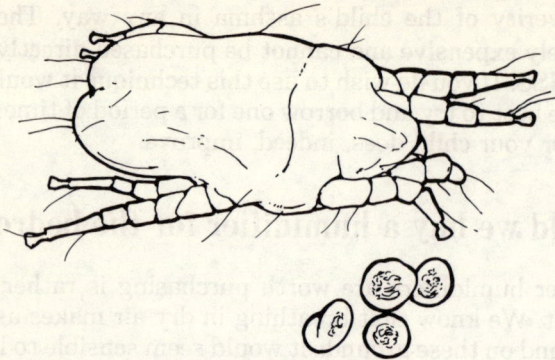

Fig. 15 The house dust mite and its 'droppings'.

find that your child has coughing and wheezing attacks if he is in the bedroom while dusting and cleaning is in progress. The house dust mite is also to some extent responsible to coughing and wheezing which occurs in the middle of the night. It would seem entirely reasonable to keep the bedroom spotlessly clean and get rid of the mites completely. With this in mind many parents have replaced

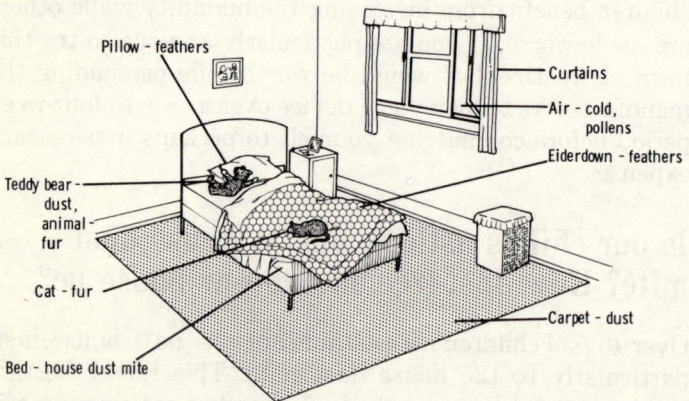

Fig. 16 Asthma-inducing items in the bedroom.

the carpets with lino-type flooring which can be cleaned more easily. Others buy blankets which can be washed every few weeks, put a layer of polythene between the mattress and the undersheet and vacuum the bedroom daily, including curtains and bedclothes. This will certainly reduce the amount of dust and house dust mite in the bedroom. Unfortunately, it is virtually impossible to eliminate the house dust mite completely and striking improvement after introducing this type of daily spring-cleaning is relatively rare. Nevertheless, it is worthwhile vacuuming the bedroom regularly (at times when your child is not present) and probably worth vacuuming the bed at the same time.

Are there any herbal remedies which can help? Are homeopathic drugs of any use?

There are some herbal remedies which have been known to relieve attacks of asthma but their effect tends to be weak and unpredictable. For this reason they cannot be recommended as alternatives to the conventional drugs we now have available. Equally, it is unlikely that your child will come to any harm if you want to try out a remedy obtained from the local herbalist. Homeopathy is a more difficult subject. It is based on a concept that if a drug can be found which produces a symptom, for example coughing, it can also be used as effective treatment if given in very dilute forms. The theory is that the remedial power of the drug increases with progressive dilution. To my knowledge there is no reputable scientific evidence that this form of treatment helps in any way, either than by suggestion. This does not mean that children with asthma will not benefit from homeopathic remedies. It is, however, only likely to occur if the child and his parents believe in the therapy. There is again no doubt that this is an entirely safe form of treatment.

Is hypnosis useful in childhood asthma?

Acute asthma can be very distressing and frightening to the child as well as to his parents. Some think that they are about to die and so it is hardly surprising that although asthmatic children are no more neurotic than their unaffected friends, emotional aspects are important. Many

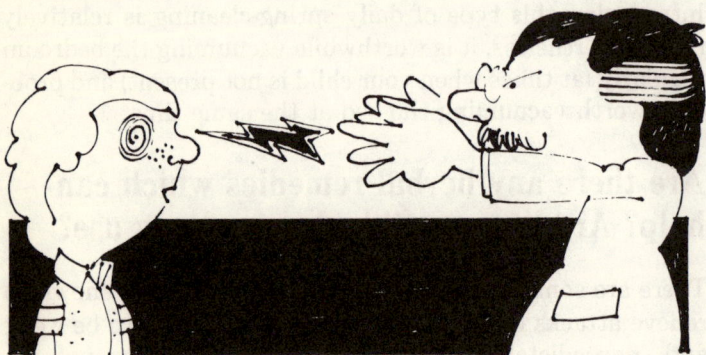

parents will notice that attacks occur more frequently at times of distress or excitement and improve as the child regains his normal composure. We have already seen that asthma does, to some extent, respond to suggestion, that there is an element of mind over body. For this reason hypnosis has been tried on many occasions. Some children have had useful improvement, particularly when taught how to induce a semi-hypnotic state in themselves, the so-called auto-suggestion. The problem is that this improvement seems to be limited to only a few children and that not all children are easily hypnotized. There is also a worry that auto-suggestion prevents the child from calling for help at times when a severe attack occurs. If you want to try hypnosis seek advice of your doctor who may either provide it himself or know a colleague who has experience with this form of treatment.

6. THE ACUTE ATTACK.

Most children with asthma are likely to have acute attacks from time to time. These are likely to be very distressing to the child. There is no doubt that the severity and length of the attack does to some extent depend upon the reaction of the parents.

What treatment should be given in an acute attack?

The drugs that are most likely to produce a rapid and dramatic end to the acute attack are the bronchodilator drugs, for example, Ventolin, Bricanyl and Alupent. Improvement usually occurs within one to two minutes if they are given by inhalation either as a powder (rotahaler), a pressurised aerosol or as a nebulised solution if you have a compressor at home. If you only have tablets or syrup, these too can be given but don't expect much improvement for 20 to 30 minutes. All these treatments work best if given very early before the lungs have filled up with secretions. There is no point in holding off starting treatment as these drugs do not lose their effect even if given frequently. They are entirely safe. If the effect from the powder or pressurised aerosol (one to three puffs) is poor, the dose can be repeated after one or two hours again without any danger. The solution inhalation can also be repeated after three hours. Sometimes when children have frequent troublesome attacks of asthma the parents will be given courses of steroids to keep at home with instructions to start these as soon as the child has a bad attack. Providing your child gets good relief from the treatment outlined above he is in no danger and can be given further bronchodilator treatment at four-hourly intervals over the next few days.

How can we stop our child panicking in the attack? How can we remain calm ourselves?

The more anxious and tense the child is the more severe will be the attack. Showing your own anxiety will not reassure the child. If you are familiar with the drugs needed, know that the drugs are always readily available and have a plan of action to cover the occasions when response to first line treatment is poor, you will feel in control and will best be able to have a calming influence on your child.

When should we seek help in an acute attack?

Usually parents have little problem in deciding whether their child is getting better or worse. What is more difficult is to decide when the attack is becoming dangerous, when extra help is required and when it is reasonable to ring the doctor or take the child up to the local hospital. The intensity of the wheezing itself can be misleading, as an increase in severity can produce an almost silent chest. It is essential that you get urgent help if your child looks in anyway blue (cyanosed) and is becoming exhausted or is no longer fully conscious. These are late signs that all is not well. It is better and safer to use the child's response to the bronchodilator drugs as the main guide. If the first and second doses of the inhaled bronchodilator drugs (Ventolin, Bricanyl and Alupent) do not produce definite improvement within a few minutes or have only a transient effect lasting for less than 60 minutes, extra treatment is essential. Your doctor may be able to re-establish control of the attack by giving an injection or starting a course of steroids. He may feel it would be safer for your child to be admitted to hospital. Many parents accept this offer with relief if they have been battling with an acute attack for some time. Most admissions to hospital are only for one to three days and cause the child very little distress.

What should we do if we cannot get hold of our own doctor in an acute attack?

Very occasionally you may find that your own doctor is understandably unavailable due to another emergency elsewhere. Asthma attacks, alas, also occur on holiday. In both these situations it is entirely reasonable to take your child up to the local hospital but first check that it has an accident and emergency department, as not all of the smaller hospitals have anyone available to cope with an acute asthma in the middle of the night. It is also worth ringing through to the hospital to let them know that you are coming. If you do not have a car or a close neighbour who can drive the family up to the hospital, dial 999, ask for the ambulance service and give clear information.

For children who have quite severe attacks special arrangements can often be made for the child to go straight up to the hospital at the beginning of an attack to get an inhalation of nebulised Ventolin or Bricanyl if this is not available at home or at the surgery or the health centre.

Could our child die in an asthma attack?

Between a half and one million children in the United Kingdom have asthma attacks at some time or another.

Fewer than 30 die each year. As a result, the chances of your child dying in an acute attack are extremely rare — considerably less than the chance that he will be killed on the roads. Investigations into these rare but tragic deaths show that those most at risk have severe chronic asthma. The risk to the child who has only occasional attacks and is entirely well in between is extremely remote. Deaths occur at home rather than in hospital, usually because the severity of the attack has not been appreciated and so appropriate treatment has not been started. The signs that all is not well have been outlined above. The child will no longer be getting relief from his bronchodilator treatment, whether this be by aerosol, inhaled powder or as nebulised salbutamol solution. He will become more and more exhausted. Children at risk look pale and there may be a blue tinge to the lips and face. Under these circumstances immediate medical help from your own doctor or from the local hospital are essential. There was a suggestion that the increase in the number of childhood asthma deaths that occurred in the 1960s was due to extensive use of inhaled bronchodilators. This is now thought to be very unlikely and that the child slipped into unconsciousness from failing to get help as response to their inhalers diminished progressively.

7. LONG TERM MANAGEMENT.

Can asthma be cured?

Although the vast majority of children should be able to lead an entirely normal and unrestrictive life, there is no evidence that any treatments we have help the child to grow out of his asthma. There are, however, some simple precautions which can modify the severity. There is, for example, little doubt that cigarette smoke does aggravate the lungs. If parents are unable to give up smoking they should ensure that they only do it away from the child.

Should we get rid of our cats/dogs/rabbits/guinea pigs/gerbils/hampsters?

This is often a difficult question to answer. If your child has attacks of wheezing and coughing, possibly also with sneezing and runny eye when coming into contact with a particular pet the answer is obviously yes. It is most unusual for the asthma to disappear completely once the pet is removed from the household, but improvement is likely. In the absence of such a situation it is more difficult to know whether the disposal of a pet will lead to sufficient benefit to compensate for the emotional disturbance which will ensue. It is sometimes worth loaning the pet to a friend or relative for several weeks to see what happens. Improvement may not be immediate as the house is likely to be heavily contaminated with the fur. The alternative is to keep the pet outside the house and thus reduce the contact.

Once a diagnosis of childhood asthma has been made it would seem foolhardy to buy any form of furry pet and run the risk of adding to the child's problems. Lack of reaction on first contact does not mean that an allergy to the animal will not develop over the next months or even years. The alternative safe pets include fish and tortoises, which sadly do not have the same attraction, and most children find these poor substitutes.

Does damp in the house make asthma worse?

This can also be a difficult question as on the one hand we know that under damp conditions both the house dust mite and mould flourish. Both are factors which produce wheezing attacks in many children. On the other hand breathing in moist air is less likely to induce wheezing than breathing in cold dry air. On the whole the balance is against damp conditions and most council housing authorities look sympathetically at requests for re-housing on the grounds that there are asthmatic children in the family, particularly if the application is accompanied by a letter from a general practitioner or hospital doctor.

Should our child take part in games at school? Are there any sports that are beneficial or harmful?

Our aim in looking after children with asthma must be to encourage them to take part in all sports along with their unaffected colleagues and friends and provide a level of treatment sufficient to allow them to compete. The occurrence of coughing and wheezing on exercise is an indication for additional therapy and not that the child should be prevented from joining in with games. Protection from exercise-induced coughing and wheezing can always almost be achieved by giving the child regular Intal or inhalations of bronchodilator drugs (for example Ventolin) immediately before the games commence, or even a combination of the two. As the airway narrowing coming on after exercise is due largely, if not entirely, to breathing in cold dry air, pretreatment is of greatest importance in the winter. Many asthmatic children find brief periods of exercise no problem and can cope with games such as football without any treatment. Prolonged exercise, such as the cross country run, presents more of a challenge but again bronchodilator inhalations at the onset can prevent wheezing even in this situation. Swimming in a heated swimming pool produces the best exercise of all. The reason for this is now apparent as the air immediately over a heated swimming pool is very humid and relatively warm, conditions which are less likely to produce wheezing.

In recent years there has been a trend to take groups of asthmatic children and to train them up, encouraged by the performance of athletes of international standing who have asthma themselves. These training programme regimes are effective. The children become more confident of their own abilities and are able to join in with more exertion before becoming breathless and starting to wheeze. Your local hospital or asthma group may well have details on a scheme in your home area.

When should we keep our child away from school?

There is no doubt that your child is more likely to pick up infections if he goes to school, that going to school on a cold windy day may bring on a mild wheezing attack, and that the emotional stresses of exams and tests can adversely affect the child's symptoms. Our aim must always be to give the asthmatic child sufficient treatment so that he can attend school on a regular basis and not miss out on his education. If your child is missing more than a few days a term through his asthma, you are either being too protective or need to have his therapy re-examined. Coughing and wheezing at night or first thing in the morning should not be considered as a reason for keeping him away from school. Providing he can get to school without difficulty and is not obviously wheezing and coughing at the time, he should be encouraged to go even if he has to miss out on games on these occasions.

Can school cope with our child's asthma?

If your child has more than very occasional asthma attacks you really must visit the school and explain the situation to the head teacher and also the form teacher. Although perhaps a little apprehensive to start with, virtually all teachers are very happy to help with the management of your child's asthma. It is often a good idea to have a spare set of medicines kept at school, either in the care of the teacher or the school nurse. This will ensure that the correct treatment is given and that the school can cope with mild wheezing attacks, so that your child can remain at school and will not be sent home unnecessarily. It will also avoid problems when your child forgets to take part of his treatment or loses it on the way to school. The teachers will want to have a clear instructions on who to contact in the event of an attack which does not settle down quickly and what to do if you are not available, whether this be to phone another relative, call your doctor or even take him to the local hospital. Careful planning of this sort can avoid people panicking and avoid unnecessary distress.

Should our child go to a special school?

For virtually all children the answer to this question is no. There are a few open air special schools which cater for children with particularly bad asthma. They are all residential and as they have to spend so much time looking after the children's ailments, educational standards tend to fall. The children who should be considered are those who spend most of their time away from school and need frequent admissions to hospital. If they respond rapidly in the hospital environment, it may be that life at home produces too many emotional and other triggers for the child to lead a normal life. Under these circumstances the possibility of transferring your child away can be considered by your doctor, the school doctor and the hospital consultant. For a small group of children there is need for such a protective environment, allowing them to gain strength, confidence and take part in class work on a regular basis. It may be that after a few terms the child could then transfer back into a normal educational system.

Should we move to another part of the country?

Parents often feel anxious and guilty that the particular place where they live may be contributing to their child's symptoms. This is almost always not the case. Often when parents move to other parts of the country the child's asthma does temporarily improve but this is rarely maintained and so the expense, inconvenience and emotional stress of loosing one's friends are not as a rule justified. Equally, if for any reason a move is necessary there are no particular guidelines on which to select where to buy a house, whether this be in the valley or on the hill side. If hay fever symptoms are a major factor with coughing and wheezing from May to July it is obviously advisable not to choose to live in the country surrounded by grass and hay!

Should we send our child to Switzerland?

It has been known for many years that some children with particularly severe asthma benefit from time spent in the Alps. Why this should be is not entirely clear but we know

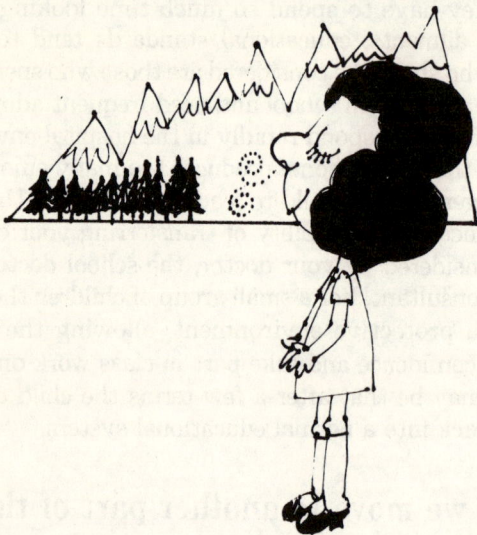

that there are virtually no mites in the dry atmosphere of the mountains. As already stated there are the occasional children who seem to thrive away from their home. This is obviously a very expensive option, not open to many families and should only be considered for those who have severe asthma with repeated admission to hospital, despite adequate treatment with steroids.

Should our child see a specialist?

The large majority of asthmatic children respond very well to treatment and do not require the specialist facilities available in the hospital. In many ways the fewer people involved in the management the better. The general practitioner who knows the child and the family well is often the best person to identify the factors responsible for a flare up of the coughing and wheezing and can then tailor the treatment to the child. The children who should be seen at the children's out-patient department or chest clinic are those with:

1. Chronic symptoms that never go away.
2. Asthma attacks which prevent the child attending school more than 90% of the time.
3. Attacks sufficiently severe to require even occasional courses of steroid tablets.

Sometimes children are referred to a specialist because there is some doubt about the diagnosis and the general practitioner considers that further investigations are required. A common and entirely acceptable reason for referral is that the parents want to be sure that their child is receiving the best treatment possible and feel that the specialist may have something to offer which their general practitioner does not. In some situations this is true. It is, for example, much easier for the hospital doctor to provide the pre-school wheezy child with a compressor and nebuliser for use at home.

Other children are referred to the specialist's out-patient clinic after a severe attack of asthma which has led to attendance at the accident and emergency department or admission to the wards. It is possible to get access into hospital system just by taking the child along to the accident and emergency department, but it is far preferable to discuss referral first with your own general practitioner who will know the most appropriate specialist to see. After your child has attended the clinic or out-patients, the specialist may feel that after one or two investigations, for example, chest X-ray, blood tests, lung function tests, only minor or no changes in therapy are required and will discharge your child back to the general practitioner. If the asthma is sufficiently difficult to manage or there are special problems further appointments may be made and then the care of your child will be shared between the hospital and your own doctor. You may find in this situation that your doctor will become reluctant to alter treatment, prefering to leave the decision to the specialist.

What should we do when we are not happy with our own general practitioner's treatment?

There is no doctor yet born who will be considered by all his patients to be entirely satisfactory and totally worthy of their confidence. Each doctor has his own way of approaching problems which is dependent upon his personality, training and experience. If his personality is very different from your own you may feel that he is not as sympathetic as you wish, that he does not take the severity of your child's symptoms sufficiently seriously, that you cannot talk to him as you would wish. Indeed it is surprising how rarely such problems arise. You may feel that you require additional advice from a specialist who will then be very happy to see your child on receiving a referral from your own doctor.If you find this support insufficient the alternative is to transfer to another doctor who suits your personality better. Friends who have children with similar problems can often give very helpful advice. You will need to register with your new chosen general practitioner but you are not under any obligation to explain the situation to your old doctor. Alternatively, you may feel that you do not have confidence in the specialist to whom you have been referred. The solution here is to discuss this with your general practitioner who will be able to arrange a transfer to another specialist, either locally or if appropriate further afield for a second opinion.

These courses of action may seem rather dramatic but confidence in your doctor and the treatment he is providing are essential if your child is going to get maximum benefit.

Why do treatments not help my baby's wheezing? Should I change the milk or diet?

Although wheezing attacks are very common in the first year of life, often following a cold, response to any form of treatment is very disappointing. Why this should be is not fully understood. Once the child is over twelve to fifteen months treatment is effective and good relief can often be provided by oral bronchodilator drugs. If this proves insufficient, regular nebulised Intal with added Ventolin or Bricanyl can lead to a dramatic improvement.

There are a few babies whose wheezing is made worse by items in the diet, particularly eggs and cow's milk. Your doctor may advise that you try changing to goat's milk or a soya substitute, although both can themselves produce allergic reactions. The number of children improving on an altered diet is small but it may be worth while trying.

8. THE PARENTS AND THE CHILD.

Although your doctor can give extensive advice the minute-to-minute decisions inevitably fall on the parents when the child is young and later on the child himself. Management is not purely giving the treatment prescribed by the doctor but involves other and more difficult decisions. For example, should your child go out today, or stay away from school? Is he fit to join in with games? Attacks of asthma can be very frightening to the parent as well as the affected child, and it is hardly surprising that fear of inducing attacks may modify the way the child is treated by other members of the family.

Should we endeavour to avoid all emotional upsets?

As I mentioned earlier, treatment should be tailored to ensure that the asthmatic child leads as normal life as possible, joining in with all the educational physical and play activities of their friends. The same applies to their emotional life. It is not possible to shield children totally from all the anxiety and stress of society, and attempts to shelter these children at home and outside from this aspect of growing up is likely to do more harm than good in the long run. The aim should be to treat your child just as you would any other non-asthmatic child, giving them love and comfort but nevertheless disciplining and chiding them when the occasions and situations arise. There are very occasional children who can bring on wheezing attacks when under this sort of pressure. This is a signal that extra help is needed, either in the form of a child specialist, or even at a child guidance clinic, as total surrender to a child's emotional blackmail will make a normal family life virtually impossible in the future and not help the child's development.

How can we reconcile our child to the treatment?

A. When very young and fighting against pills, medicines and face masks.
B. When growing older and feeling that treatment is an unnecessary evil, or even 'infra dig.'

As is implied in these questions children are most reluctant to accept treatment as toddlers and teenagers. Very young children will usually take medicine providing the taste is acceptable to them. If your child repeatedly refuses a preparation discuss this with your doctor as it is very likely that there is an alternative which will prove more satisfactory. Sometimes small tablets, for example, steroids, have to be prescribed. If these are a problem check with your doctor whether these can be crushed, as they then can be camouflaged in jam or honey. If you need to resort to this for more than a short time, give the treatments immediately before meals to reduce the risk of dental caries. Regular tooth brushing after meals will further limit any unnecessary damage.

Not all young children take to face masks and nebulisers, although it is surprising how quickly even children of one to two years appreciate the benefit they get and ask for treatment as asthma attacks come on. Familiarity with the device is undoubtedly helpful. Don't be worried about wasting several doses by leaving it running near your child in order to gain his confidence. Combining the treatment with a story or television programme also helps. If there is a total refusal don't fight but try again two to three weeks later. With this approach it is rare for young children not to be happy to accept this somewhat tedious but highly effective form of therapy.

The teenagers with their rather fatalistic bravado attitudes are harder to deal with and create a great deal of stress within the family. Parents often find that parental pressure works adversely and that the child refuses his treatment 'to spite them'. Usually the children will continue to use bronchodilators drugs when wheezing becomes a problem but omit or forget to take regular therapy, including Intal, Theophylline and steroids. Your doctor or specialist is likely to have some influence. He may also be able to reach a compromise and simplify the treatment as far as possible so that regular medication only need to be taken at night and morning when friends and colleagues are not around.

How can we cope with the lack of sleep and our own irritability?

Asthma is often at its worst during the night, particularly in the under-5s. Many parents find that it is difficult to cope working all day and then having to spend most of the night trying to comfort their child. Sometimes the child sleeps through but coughs repeatedly, keeping other members of the family awake. Chronic tiredness and sense of frustration can make the parents irritable and less sympathetic to the child's distress creating a vicious circle. At the far extreme is a feeling that you must somehow stop your child's endless coughing, even if this means hitting the child, throwing him

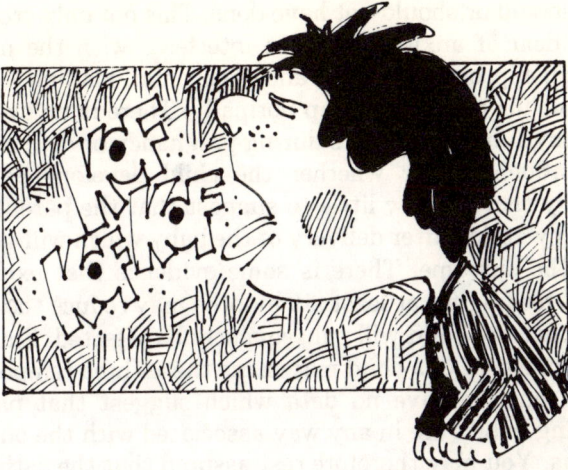

against ·a wall or smothering him with a pillow. These thoughts are not uncommon even though they seem horrific to those who have not experienced them. They are an indication for seeking immediate help. In all these situations the first step is to get further medical advice as it is almost always possible to prevent continuous nightly coughing, even if symptoms still break through for a few days when the child has a cold or when going through a stressful period. At these times it is reasonable for the night vigil to be shared among the family. If the problem becomes critical and you are worried that you may do your asthmatic child physical harm you should immediately contact your doctor or take the baby up to the hospital so that he can be admitted, partly to sort out the asthma but also to provide you with a needed rest so that you can regain control of the situation.

Is asthma due to any neglect on our part? Is our child's asthma our fault?

Many parents have feelings of guilt about their child's asthma, worrying that this has arisen from something that they should or should not have done. This not only creates a great deal of anxiety but also interferes with the normal relationship between them and their child, making it more difficult for him to grow up normally. There is no evidence that anything that occurs during pregnancy or delivery has any influence over whether the child develops asthma. Equally there is now little to suggest that the parents can take any action after delivery of the baby which will greatly alter the outcome. There is some evidence that exclusive breast feeding for at least six months may reduce the likelihood that the child will subsequently be affected. Smoking in the presence of a child may make the asthma temporarily worse, but we have no data which suggest that parents smoking habits are in any way associated with the onset of asthma. You may therefore rest assured that the asthma is not your fault and that guilt feelings are not only unjustified but are positively unhelpful to your growing child.

If there is asthma on both sides of the family should we have children?

A strong family history of asthma does increase the risk that children will have asthma. The increase is, however, not very great and certainly should not influence whether you should have children or not. Severity of asthma does not run in the family, so that even if there are relatives on both sides of the family who have particularly severe attacks the chances are very much in favour of any asthma being relatively mild and easy to treat.

Having a child with troublesome asthma can place large stresses and burdens upon the immediate relatives and for this reason some parents elect not to enlarge their families further. There can be no guarantee that the next child will not have asthma, but again the chances are against it.

Can we get more support?

You may feel that a trouble shared is a trouble halved, and there are now local asthma groups that help in various parts of the country. These provide social occasions where parents with asthmatic children get together, discuss their problems and worries and find out how others have coped in similar situations. These groups have access to more information on childhood asthma and often arrange for talks to be given by experts on the care of the children with asthma. The groups also have an important role raising money for nebulisers for families with young asthmatic children and also providing extremely valuable support for research into the causes and management of childhood asthma.

Can we get financial support to help the family?

If your child is over the age of two years and has such difficult asthma that you have to get up frequently during the night, you may be entitled to a night attendance allowance. This should be applied for from the local social services department. The awarding of this allowance is by no means automatic and the social services authority will require a report from a medical officer who will visit and interview you at home. The payment is in recognition that you are unable to lead a normal life with the family and the concept behind the payment is that with it you will be able to pay others to help to look after your child at home.

9. THE FUTURE.

Will my child grow out of his asthma?

All parents ask this question which is unfortunately impossible to answer completely. Wheezing is at its most common in the first five years of life. Nearly half of these children will either stop wheezing or have much less trouble by the time they are five to seven years old. What we cannot do at present is identify the children who will show this trend. By and large those with severe asthma are least likely to improve. Children wheezing after acute bronchiolitis, the severe viral infection which usually occurs in the first few months of life, often do not have any evidence of allergic problems. These children are particularly likely to improve but again it is not possible to predict in advance whether this will happen. Asthma can show an improvement at any time during childhood but the next most common time for attacks to subside is during puberty. Again, approximately half the children will improve very considerably, often losing their symptoms completely. Those with severe asthma improve the least again. Long term studies have shown that unfortunately a number of children who grow out of their problems in adolescence will have further wheezing five to ten years later. This has obvious implications for career advice.

Is there anything we can do to ensure that our child grows out of his asthma?

There are no treatments however effective they are at relieving and controlling symptoms which appear to alter the long term course of asthma. There are two steps which may make a difference. It would seem reasonable not to introduce any hair or fur coated pets in to the family. These may not produce problems in the short term but allergies may develop later. Equally, smoking should be avoided in the presence of the child if at all possible. There is no doubt that cigarette smoke is irritant to asthmatic children. In addition there is good evidence that if the child himself smokes this will have a strong tendency to make any persisting asthma a great deal more severe. The adverse and potentially dangerous effects of smoking should be instilled into the child from a relatively young age.

If our child grows out of his asthma what is the chance of it returning?

It is only in recent years that there have been any studies into the long term outcome of childhood asthma. We so far know that the trend towards improvement that occurs throughout childhood tends to run out in the late teenage years and by the early twenties some people get their symptoms of coughing and wheezing back. How frequently this occurs we do not yet know, nor do we know whether further relapses will occur with any frequency in the next decade. The overall risk is not likely to be high in view of the relative frequency of wheezing in childhood compared to adults.

How can we help our asthmatic child grow into adult life? Should he manage his own drugs?

As has already been stated it is vitally important for the asthmatic child to lead as normal as life as possible, joining in with all activities of his unaffected peers and not to be isolated and over-protected. As he grows older he will be able to take over the management of his drugs, and he should certainly be doing this by the time he is a teenager. It will remain important for you to keep an unobtrusive eye over him to ensure that his asthma control is not deteriorating progressively due to the under-use of therapy.